Pedro Djacir Escobar Martins

Use of stem cells in skin healing

Pedro Djacir Escobar Martins

Use of stem cells in skin healing

Adult adipose tissue stem cells in skin healing

ScienciaScripts

Imprint

Any brand names and product names mentioned in this book are subject to trademark, brand or patent protection and are trademarks or registered trademarks of their respective holders. The use of brand names, product names, common names, trade names, product descriptions etc. even without a particular marking in this work is in no way to be construed to mean that such names may be regarded as unrestricted in respect of trademark and brand protection legislation and could thus be used by anyone.

Cover image: www.ingimage.com

This book is a translation from the original published under ISBN 978-613-9-64124-6.

Publisher:
Sciencia Scripts
is a trademark of
Dodo Books Indian Ocean Ltd. and OmniScriptum S.R.L publishing group

120 High Road, East Finchley, London, N2 9ED, United Kingdom
Str. Armeneasca 28/1, office 1, Chisinau MD-2012, Republic of Moldova, Europe
Printed at: see last page
ISBN: 978-620-7-74269-1

To my wife Rejane for her constant encouragement and co-operation.

To my children Marjory, Pedro Alexandre and Carlos Henrique and my grandchildren Mariana, Enrico and Catarina, who are extensions of my life.

To my parents João and Ecilda (in memoriam) because they taught me the first ways to get here.

To my late first wife Yvonne (in memoriam), mother of my children.

ACKNOWLEDGEMENTS

To Prof. Dr Jefferson Braga da Silva for his guidance and support during the completion of this thesis.To Prof. Dr Denise Cantarelli Machado for her encouragement and guidance in the area of cell biology.

To Prof Dr Vinicius Duval for his guidance and encouragement in photometric evaluations.

To Prof. Dr Mario Wagner for his guidance in the statistical analyses of this thesis.

To Prof Dr Lucio Bakos for his kindness in participating as an evaluator of this research.

To Prof Rinaldo de Angeli Pinto for his kindness in participating as an evaluator of this research.

To Dr Antonio Pinto for his kindness in participating as an evaluator in this research.

To Dr Alexandre Vonbel Padoin for his support and collaboration.

To Dr Marcelo Marafon Maino for his support and collaboration.

To the Residents and Preceptors of the Plastic Surgery Service at HSL-PUCRS for their support and understanding.

To the librarian Rosária Maria Lucia Prenna Geremia for her support and goodwill.

To the patients who underwent this study.

SUMMARY

Introduction: Surgery will achieve all its objectives if, in addition to the other results, the skin scar looks good, especially in plastic surgery. Studies carried out on foetuses undergoing surgery in utero have shown that, after birth, the scars were minimal or imperceptible. There is evidence that there is less inflammation and less collagen accumulation in foetal healing compared to adults. These facts instigate the possibilities of manipulating skin continuity solutions in adults. Plastic surgeons, in particular, have turned their attention to skin healing. In their interventions, they use procedures and therapies or cosmetic measures to make scars less noticeable.

Patients and Methods: This was a randomised controlled study with the aim of evaluating skin healing after the implantation of adult adipose tissue stem cells. Eighteen patients from the Plastic Surgery Service at HSL-PUCRS were selected, taking into account inclusion and exclusion criteria. The stem cells used were autologous, extracted from adipose tissue in the infraumbilical region before abdominoplasty in the selected patients. The adult stem cells extracted from adipose tissue before skin synthesis were infiltrated into the dermis of the surgical wound in the suprapubic region. The post-operative evaluation was carried out using the Draaijers scale by three blinded medical evaluators and by the patients themselves by self-assessment. Photometric evaluation was also carried out using digital photography.

Results: Of the 18 patients operated on, 17 had excellent or good results (94%) and 1 who had suture dehiscence was considered to have a poor result (5.5%). Another 5 patients were excluded due to abandonment during the study (27%), leaving 12 (66.6%) at the end. No statistically significant difference was found when comparing the photometric aspects. When comparing the patients' assessments, 6 aspects were considered (pain, itching, colour, stiffness, thickness and irregularity). Considering all the evaluation events over the observation period, 42 measurement points were obtained. In these, a significance level of $P = 0.12$ was reached in favour of the stem cell intervention. In the medical observers' assessment, 5 aspects were considered (vascularisation, pigmentation, thickness, contracture and elasticity). When the distribution of evaluations over the observation period was considered, 35 measurement points were obtained. In these, a significance level of P = 0.003 was reached in favour of the stem cell intervention. Considering all the evaluations carried out by doctors, patients and photometry, a statistically significant difference was found in favour of implantation with adult adipose tissue stem cells, $p<0.001$.

Conclusion: The results of skin healing in a post-operative abdominoplasty wound after the implantation of adult stem cells derived from adipose tissue were satisfactory.

Keywords: Stem cells. Healing. Abdominoplasty.

SUMMARY

CHAPTER 1

INTRODUCTION

Since the time of the Egyptians, surgeons have been concerned with wounds and their healing, as evidenced in the papyri of Edwin S. Smith (Porter R, 1997). The closure of the surgical wound is a basic condition for successful surgery. Knowledge of the healing process is essential for the doctor to be able to manipulate the tissues properly in order to achieve an ideal result.

The healing phases are divided into inflammatory, proliferative and maturation (Sabiston Textbook of Surgery, 2004; Lorenz PA, Longaker MT, 2006). When the injury occurs, the inflammatory or reactive phase begins, in which the body's defences are directed towards reacting to the action of the trauma and limiting the amount of damage. This phase lasts around 4 days. The proliferative or regenerative phase, which begins on the fourth day, lasts approximately 14 days. This is the process of repair through re-epithelialisation, which is the synthesis of the connective tissue matrix, and neovascularisation, to relieve the ischaemia caused by the trauma. The maturation or remodelling phase is the period when the scar contracts due to collagen interlacing, shrinkage and a reduction in oedema. This is the longest phase of healing, starting around the eighth day and lasting until the sixth month or more. The tension of the scar increases rapidly within a period of 1 to 6 weeks and reaches its maturation plateau after around 1 year. All three phases can occur simultaneously, but they last for different lengths of time. At certain times, the processes of each phase can become confused.

In such a complex set of events, various factors can interfere with the healing process and its evolution, such as infection, local tissue ischaemia, diabetes mellitus, radiation, malnutrition, exogenous medication and mineral and vitamin deficiencies (Lorenz PA, Longaker MT, 2006).

The scar can be considered adequate, inadequate or proliferative (Figures 1, 2, 3 and 4). These results are determined by the synthesis of collagen and the balance of its degradation. If this balance tilts in either direction, the result will not be satisfactory. In chronic open wounds, there is greater inflammation, with more collagen degradation than synthesis. The opposite occurs in proliferative scars, hypertrophic scars and keloids, where collagen deposition exceeds degradation (Lorenz PA, Longaker MT, 2006).

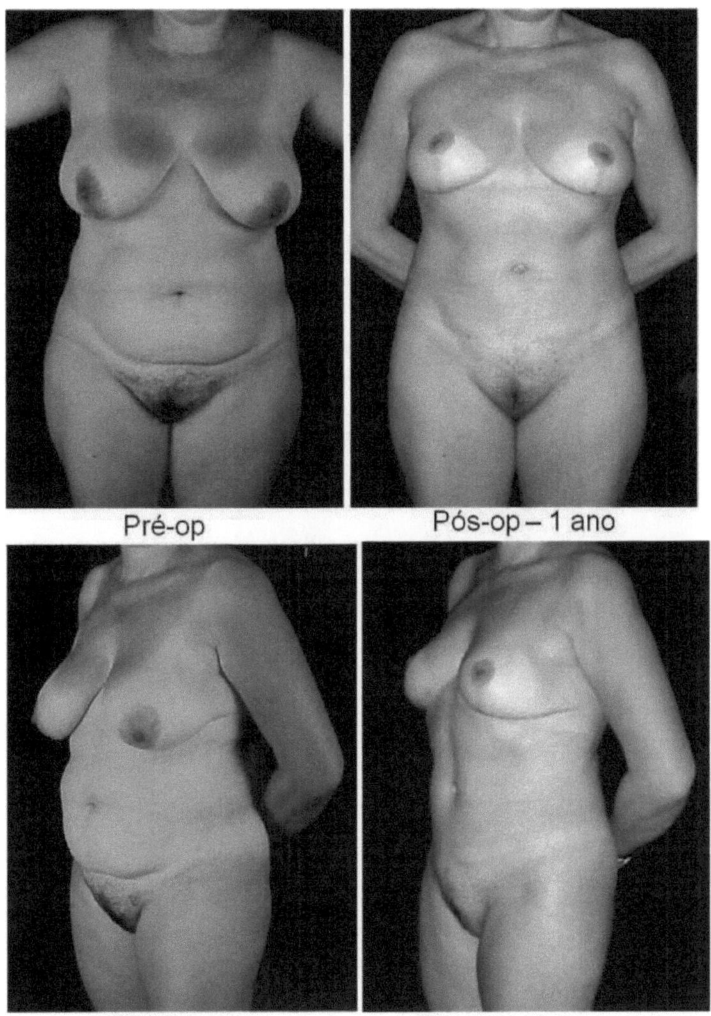

Figure 1 - Adequate healing on the skin of the abdomen and breasts.

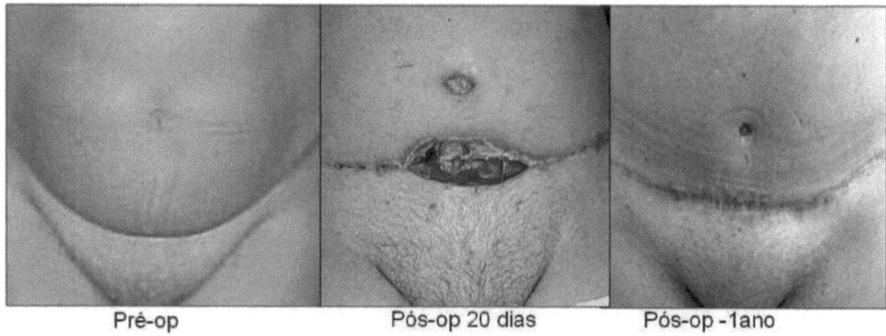

Figura 2   - Inadequate healing of the abdominal skin due to necrosis and suture dehiscence and

healing by second intention.

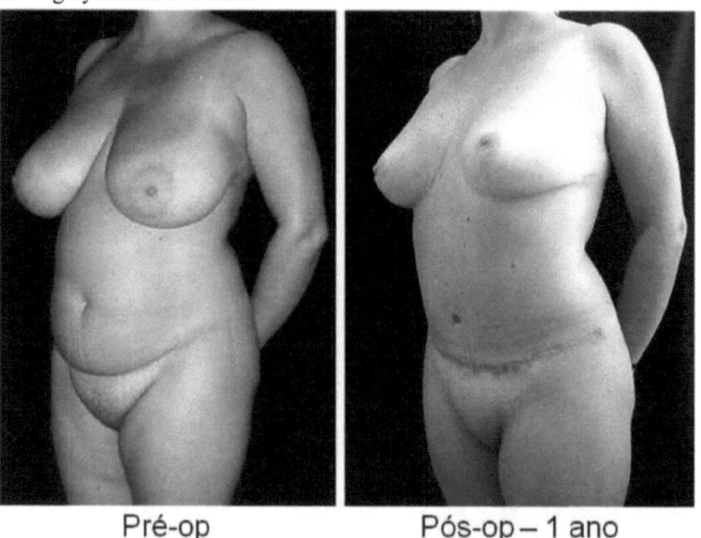

Figura 3   - Same patient as in Figure 2. Inadequate scarring on the skin of the abdomen and

adequate on the breasts.

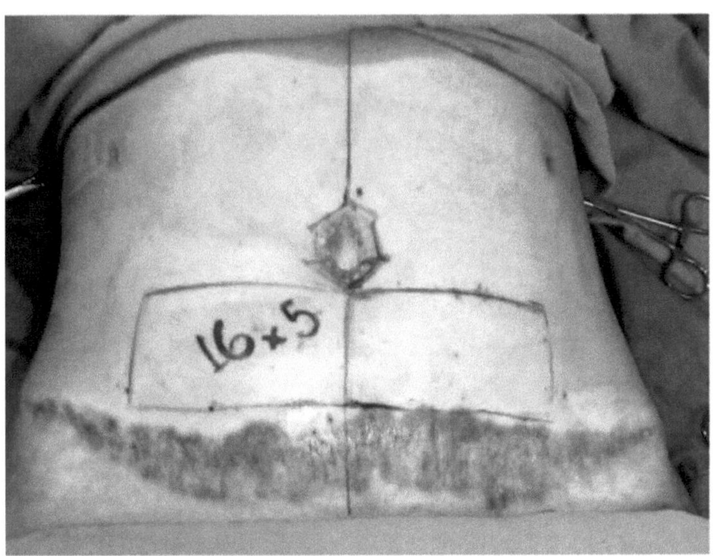

Figura 4   - Proliferative scarring in abdominoplasty.

Studies on wound healing in human foetuses that were operated on in utero showed that after birth the scars were minimal or even imperceptible. The younger the foetus at the time of the surgical procedure, the more likely it was that the scar would not be visible (Adzick NS, Longaker MT, 1992). Lin (Lin R, Sullivan K, Argenta P, et al, 1994) concluded that foetal fibroblasts remained faithful to their phenotypes, even when transplanted into adults. This scarring process develops in the absence of inflammation in the repairs, resulting in a non-apparent scar. According to Estes (Estes JM, Vande Berg JS, Adzick NS, et al 1994), the fibroblasts of the foetal wound do not develop a state of activation (myofibroblasts) until late in gestation. Bullard (Bullard M, Cass D, Adzick N, Banda M, 1996) showed that dermal fibroblasts present much more significant interstitial collagenase in foetal wounds than in adult wounds. There is evidence that there is less inflammation and a reduction in collagen accumulation in foetal healing compared to adult healing. These facts raise the possibility of manipulating the solution of skin continuity in the adult, with the aim of limiting the intensity of the inflammatory process and thus obtaining a better result in the scar.

Plastic surgeons, in particular, focus their attention on skin healing. In their surgical interventions, they try to conceal the scars, positioning them according to the lines of force of the skin, in places where they cannot be seen or where they are minimally perceptible. When the scars are located in constantly exposed places, such as on the face, for example, they use therapeutic and cosmetic behaviours or measures to conceal them, with the aim of making them less noticeable (Lorenz PA, Longaker MT, 1994; Xiao Z, Zhang F, Cui Z, 2009; Horswell BB, 1998; Viera MH, Amini S, Barman B, 2009; HaedersdalM, Moreau KE, Beyer DM, Nymann P, Alsbj0rn, 2009).

Progress in cell and molecular biology studies could have a major impact on understanding the healing process and its clinical application.

CHAPTER 2

THEORETICAL FRAMEWORK

2.1 STEM CELLS

Stem cell research is improving our understanding of how an organism develops from a single cell (blastula) and how damaged cells are replaced by healthy cells in adult organisms (Daley GQ, Goodell MA , Snyder EY, 2003; Fodor WL, 2003). This replacement process is an area of intense academic and applied research. This area of science, based on the use of stem cells to treat diseases, is known as regenerative medicine (Fodor WL, 2003) and has evolved greatly. Stem cells are fundamental not only for coordinating the formation of organs from the embryonic stage to the adult individual, but also for their important role in tissue regeneration and repair. The main characteristics of these cells are their capacity for self-renewal and differentiation into multiple cell lineages. Although there are numerous criteria proposed to define what stem cells are, in short, they must be undifferentiated cells capable of proliferation, self-renewal, production of numerous functionally differentiated cells and tissue regeneration after injury (Loeffler M, Bratke T, Paulus U, 1997). There are three main types of stem cells, which are classified according to their tissue of origin: (I) embryonic stem cells, derived from the inner layer of cells in the blastocyst; (II) umbilical cord stem cells, present in umbilical cord blood; and (III) bone marrow stem cells, located in the bone marrow stroma. The latter, together with those located in adult tissues such as adipose, neural and muscular tissue, are also called adult stem cells.

From a therapeutic point of view, i.e. in terms of their application or tissue engineering (TE), the different stem cells have advantages and disadvantages. Due to the practical difficulties of obtaining embryonic stem cells, considering ethical and legal aspects, most researchers have carried out their studies with adult stem cells, mainly those derived from bone marrow stroma (Pittenger MF, Mackay AM, Beck SC et al, 1999; Tuan RS, Boland G, Tuli R, 2003; Tohill M, Terenghi G, 2004; Braga-Silva J, et al, 2009). More recent studies have shown that this cell population can also be isolated from adipose tissue (Martinez- Estrada OM, Munoz-Santos Y, Julve J, et al, 2005; Zuk PA,

Zhu M, Mizumo H, et al, 2003; De Ugarte DA, Morizono K, Elbarbar A, et al, 2003; Safford KM, Hicok KC, Safford SD, et al, 2002), collected through liposuction (Illouz YG, 1980; Fournier P, 1983) (Figure 5). Some authors prefer not to use the term stem cells and refer to this adipose tissue material as processed lipoaspirate (PLA) cells or adipose-derived adult stem cells (ADAS) (Zuk PA, Zhu M, Mizumo H, et al, 2003; De Ugarte DA, Morizono K, Elbarbar A, et al, 2003; Fraser JK, Wulur I, Alfonso Z, Hedrick MH, 2006; Lambert APFandonai AF, Bonatto D, Machado DC, Henriques JAP, 2009). The ease with which they can be obtained encourages research into controlled studies with autologous adult stem cells extracted from adipose tissue.

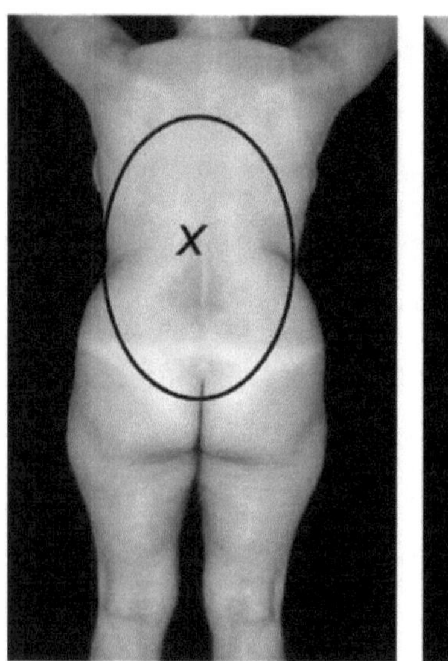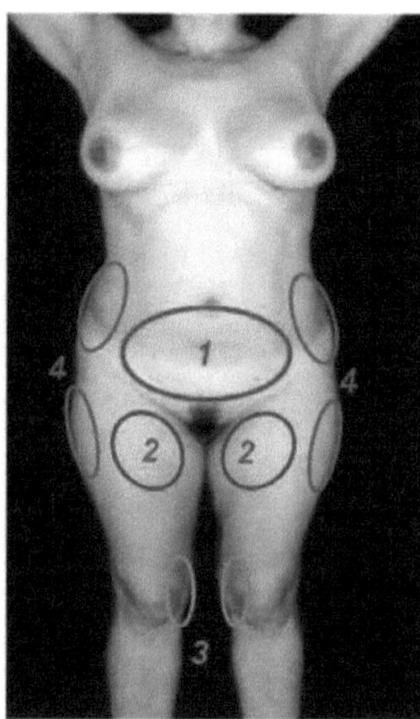

Figura 5   - Regions of the body contour where liposuction is most commonly performed and which could be stem cell donor zones. In this study, area no. 1 (infraumbilical) was chosen.

2.2 ABDOME

Since ancient times, human beings have paid special attention to their own bodies, as can be clearly seen in early works of art: the Venus of Willendorf (Figure 6) is considered by many to be the oldest sculptural representation of the human form; the Venus of Laussel (Figure 7) is considered to be the symbol of fertility. In these sculptures, it can be seen that, at that time, the breasts and abdomen were given greater importance than the face, perhaps because they were parts of the body linked to reproduction.

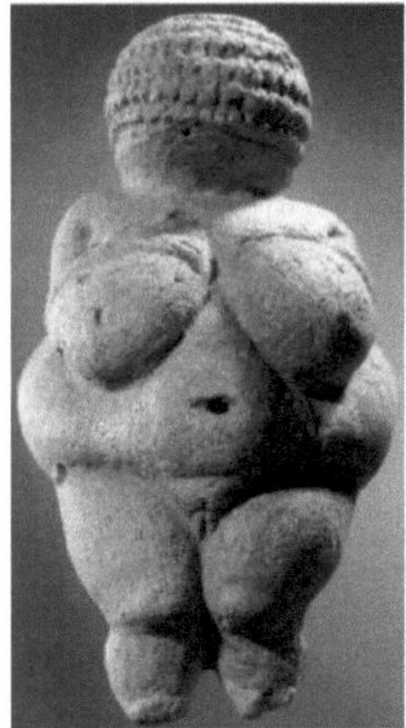
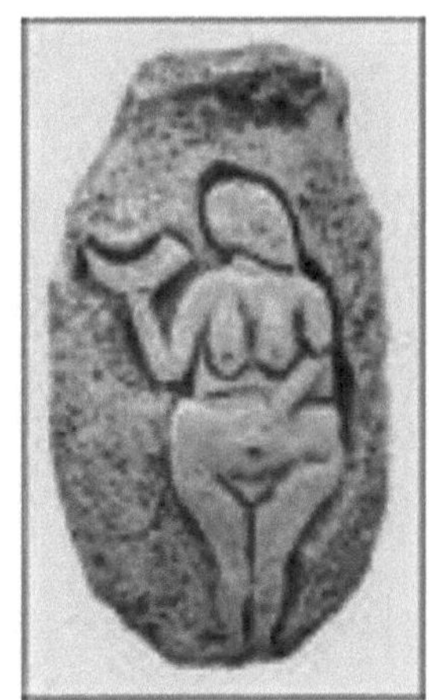

Figure 6 - Willendorf's Venus: the abdomen, genitals and breasts are well emphasised, while the face lacks detail. Source: Willendorf windows photo gallery

Figure 7 - Lausell's Venus: abdomen and pelvis are well emphasised and the face is neglected..Source:en.wikipedia.org/wiki/laussel's_venus

The abdomen is the focus of many complaints from patients who consult plastic surgeons. Due to its location, changes in shape and volume can lead to alterations in body contour. They often cause functional disturbances, with repercussions especially for the spine. Abdominal protrusion is usually associated with adiposity, sagging skin and the musculo-aponeurotic wall, either alone or together. The aim of abdominoplasty is to resect excess infraumbilical dermoadipose and reposition the structures of the musculo-aponeurotic wall of the abdomen.

There is a huge variety of techniques that address the abdominal wall. In 1890, Demars performed an infraumbilical transverse dermolipectomy. Since then, there have been countless other surgical procedures to treat abdominal lipodystrophies (Sinder R., 2005).

In this study, abdominoplasty was performed, which consists of detaching the dermoadipose panicle, in the juxta-aponeurotic plane, from a suprapubic transverse incision to the xiphoid appendix and ribs. After treating the muscle-aponeurotic wall and repositioning the umbilicus, the flap is pulled inferiorly. After drying out the excess dermoadipose, the flap is sutured in the lower suprapubic

13

incision. The steps of this procedure, with some personal tactics, are described in several important books for training plastic surgeons (Pitman GH, 1997; Pitanguy I, 1981; Vasconez LO, De La Torre JI, 2006; Pontes R, 2004).

Liposuction is often combined with abdominoplasty techniques to remove localised excess fat (Pontes R, 2004). The fact that these two procedures can be combined in the same surgical procedure, with obvious advantages for patients, was ideal for the study carried out.

CHAPTER 3

OBJECTIVE

To evaluate skin healing in a post-operative abdominoplasty wound after the implantation of adult stem cells derived from adipose tissue.

CHAPTER 4

PATIENTS AND METHODS

4.1 DELINEATION

Randomised controlled trial.

4.2 PATIENTS

Eighteen patients were selected from the Plastic Surgery Department of the São Lucas Hospital at PUCRS. All the abdominoplasties were performed by the same surgeon between August and September 2007 and met the criteria described below.

4.2.1 Inclusion criteria

- Patients at the Plastic Surgery Service of the São Lucas Hospital of PUCRS who had an indication for abdominoplasty.
- White skin.
- Female.
- Aged between 30 and 45, with children.
- No stretch marks in the supraumbilical region.
- BMI - 20 to 26.

4.2.2 Exclusion criteria

T Smoking.

- History of hypertrophic scars or keloids.

- Diabetes mellitus.

- Any pathology of the skin or connective tissue.

- Previous supraumbilical scar.

- Supraumbilical striae.

- BMI - outside the parameters

- Prolonged use of corticosteroids.

- Previous chemotherapy or radiotherapy.

- Post-weight loss in obesity.

- Infection.

- Haematoma.

- Seroma.

- Dehiscence after abdominoplasty.

- Patient giving up during the study.

4.3 Obtaining adult stem cells from adipose tissue

The extraction of adult stem cells from adipose tissue was carried out at the Cell Therapy Centre of the Biomedical Research Institute of PUCRS, as follows: 20 mL of adipose tissue were divided into two tubes and washed with 40 mL of DPBS *(Dullbecco's phosphate buffered saline; Invitrogen Corp., Carlsbad, CA, USA)*, containing 2% (v/v) foetal bovine serum (FBS; Invitrogen Corp., Carlsbad, CA, USA) to remove the red blood cells. The suspension was centrifuged at 450 x g for 5 minutes. The adipose tissue was transferred to a new tube in which 0.015% (w/v) collagenase (Sigma Co., St. Louis, MO, USA) diluted in DPBS was added to a total of 50 mL. The tube was placed on an orbital shaker and incubated at 37°C for 45 minutes until the tissue was completely dissociated. The collagen was inactivated with DMEM culture medium (Dulbecco's modified eagle medium; Invitrogen Corp., Carlsbad, CA, USA), containing 10% (v/v) FBS (Invitrogen Corp., Carlsbad, CA, USA), and the solution was divided into two tubes. The cells were centrifuged at 1,200 x g for 10 minutes and the supernatant was discarded. The cells were resuspended with 10 mL of DPBS containing 10% (v/v) FBS, followed by centrifugation for washing. The total number of cells was then quantified on a haemocytometer. The cells were resuspended in saline at a density of 5×10^8 cells per mL for infiltration into the scar.

Flow cytometry was performed with the following antibodies: CD73, CD105 and CD117. The samples were analysed on a FACScalibur flow cytometer (Becton Dickinson Immunocytometry Systems, San Jose, CA, USA). An aliquot of 100 pL of the suspension of adult adipose tissue stem cells was used to characterise the cell populations. 20 pL of each antibody was added and the solution was incubated at room temperature for 30 minutes in the dark. The sample was centrifuged at 200 x g for 5 minutes and the supernatant was discarded. The sample was washed with 2 mL of PBS (PBS, 0.1% sodium azide and 1% FBS) by centrifugation at 200 x g for 5 minutes. The supernatant was discarded and the cells were resuspended with 500 pL of PBS.

4.4 Use of adult stem cells from adipose tissue

Only cells obtained from autologous adipose tissue were used in the patients in this study. Their implantation did not cause any changes to the surgical sequence or a significant increase in the duration of the proposed procedure.

The adipose tissue was collected a maximum of 5 minutes before starting the abdominoplasty. The implantation of adipose tissue stem cells had a similar duration. The separation of these adipose tissue cells was carried out simultaneously with the surgery, with a similar duration to the abdominoplasty.

All the patients who took part in this study were operated on by the same surgeon. They all underwent the same surgical technique (Vasconez LO, De La Torre JI, 2006; Pontes R, 2004), which consisted of liposuction of the infraumbilical region followed by abdominoplasty. These two procedures, because they were carried out in the same surgical procedure, made it easier to produce the scar that is the subject of this research and to obtain the adipose tissue from which the adult stem cells were taken.Before starting the abdominoplasty, 30 mL of adipose tissue was collected from the infraumbilical region, where there is a high concentration of adult stem cells (Padoin AV, Braga-Silva J, Martins P, et al, 2008). Liposuction was performed using a 50 mL disposable syringe, a 4 millimetre gauge cannula and a 25 centimetre length. To avoid any changes to the adipose tissue, this procedure was carried out without any infiltration at the site (dry procedure) (Fournier P, 1983). In the syringe itself, under sterile conditions, this adipose tissue was sent to the Cell Therapy Centre of the PUCRS Biomedical Research Institute to extract the adult stem cells while the surgery was carried out.

4.5 SURGICAL TECHNIQUE

4.5.1 Anaesthesia

All the patients were operated on under epidural anaesthesia, with a puncture in the intercostal space at the L3-L4 level. 150 mg of 0.75% ropivacaine hydrochloride and 100 mg of fentanyl citrate were injected into the epidural space. During the operation, the patient was sedated with midazolam 15 mg intravenously (IV) in fractioned doses.

4.5.2 Liposuction

Before starting the abdominoplasty, liposuction was performed in the infraumbilical region and adipose tissue was collected to separate the adult stem cells. In all cases, a technique described by Fournier (Fournier P, 1983) was used, which consists of dry syringe liposuction, i.e. without any infiltration. The cannula connected to the syringe is inserted into the site to be liposuctioned. The plunger of the syringe is pulled and clamped in order to create negative pressure for the procedure (Figure 8).

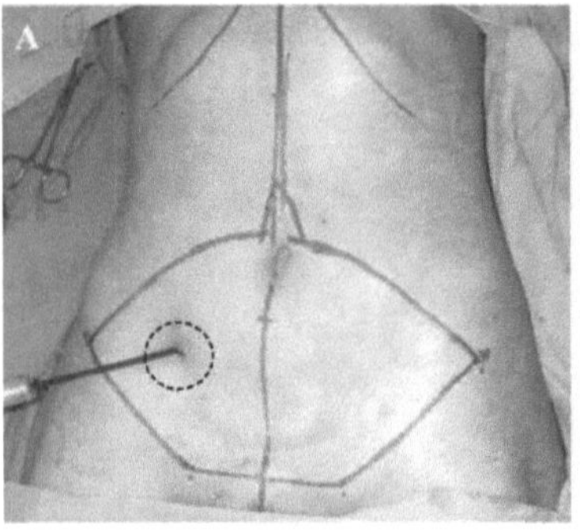
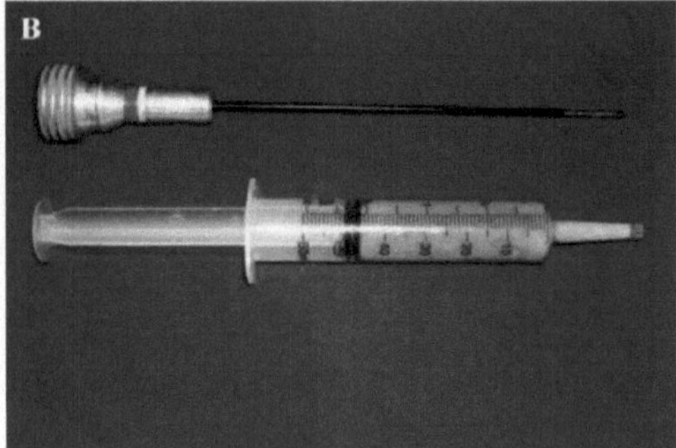

Figure 8 - Liposuction with a syringe.

A) Demarcation of the flap of skin and subcutaneous tissue to be resected (the liposuction cannula inserted into the flap can be seen in the detail).

B) Liposuction cannula and syringe with adipose tissue to be sent to IPB/PUCRS.

4.5.3 Abdominoplasty

The abdominoplasty followed the same surgical sequence in all cases. Prior resection of the skin and subcutaneous tissue flap of the infraumbilical region in the area extending from the umbilical scar to the pubic region, situated between the two anterior superior iliac spines (Vasconez LO, De La Torre JI, 2006; Pontes R, 2004) (Figure 9). Next, the supraumbilical dermogordurotic flap was detached to the level of the ribs and the xiphoid appendix. The muscle-aponeurotic wall of the abdomen was then repositioned by plication using separate stitches of mononylon 2.0 (Ethicon[®]). The umbilical scar was fixed with 4.0 mononylon stitches (Ethicon[®]) on the muscle-aponeurotic wall and sutured with the same thread to the skin of the supraumbilical dermoadipose flap that had been pulled to the pubic edge of the incision.

in its new position. To complete the abdominoplasty, the upper and lower edges of the surgical wound were synthesised in all planes. This synthesis will result in the abdominoplasty scar, on which the stem cell research was carried out (Figure 10).

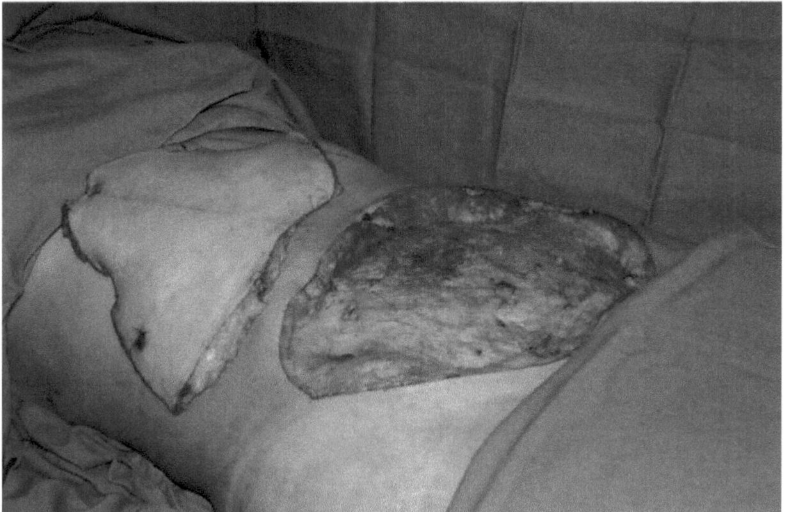

Figura 9   - Resected flap before supraumbilical detachment (Pontes R, 2004).

The skin was always sutured using the same method, i.e. 4.0 mononylon thread (Ethicon®) in the subdermal layer and 3.0 mononylon thread (Ethicon®) in the subcutaneous cellular tissue and intradermal layer. In all patients, a 1/4 suction drain (Drenoplass®) was placed through a lower counterincision in the pubic region. The purpose of this drainage was to avoid collections that could distend the skin and alter the tension on the suture lines at the research site.

4.6 IMPLANTING ADULT STEM CELLS FROM ADIPOSE TISSUE INTO THE SKIN

To carry out this study, the segment located in the suprapubic region, at the site of the abdominoplasty scar, was selected, marking 5 centimetres on each side of the midline (Figure 10). The implantation of adult adipose tissue stem cells was randomised in relation to the sides, without the knowledge of the patients or the observers.

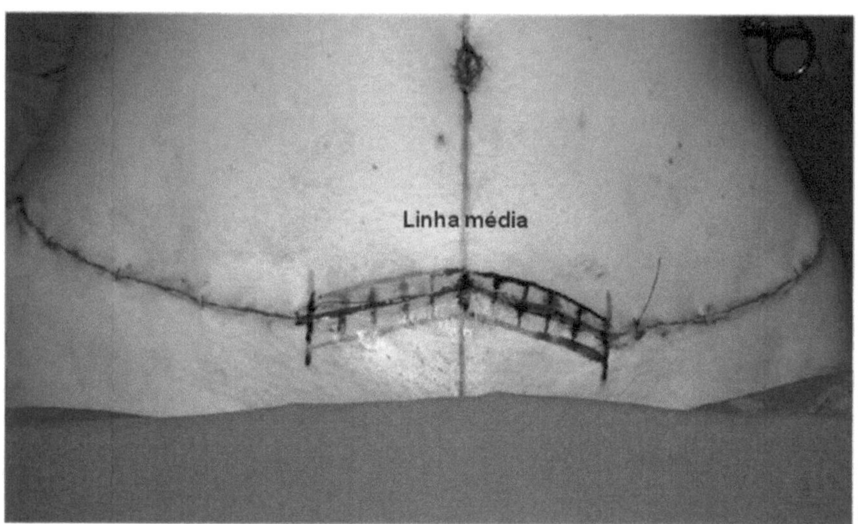

Figura 10   - Abdominoplasty surgical wound, before the final suture in the suprapubic region. Area demarcated at the site of stem cell implantation in the dermis. The implant sides were randomised in relation to the midline.

Before the skin was synthesised, the stem cells suspended in saline were implanted into the dermis of the surgical wound. The volume needed to cover 1 cm^2 of the skin surface was previously calculated by injecting methylene blue into the dermis, which was 0.5 mL (Figures 11 and 12). On the randomised side, 5 mL of saline was injected into both edges of the surgical wound, containing adult adipose tissue stem cells at a density of $5x10^8$ per mL[18] . On the contralateral side, which served as a control, the same volume of saline solution was injected. In this way, it was possible to compare the evolution of healing in the same patient with and without the implantation of adult adipose tissue stem cells.

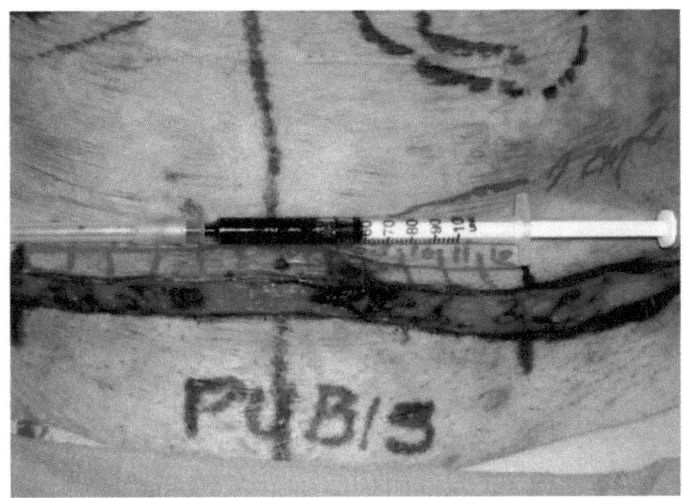

Figura 11   - Intradermal infiltration with methylene blue to calculate the volume needed to cover 1cm^2 of the skin.

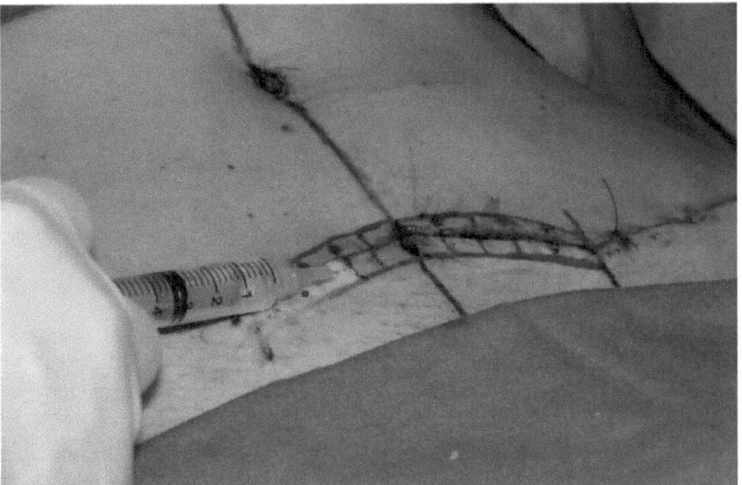

Figura 12   - Intradermal implantation of stem cells (0.5% mL/cm^2), on the control side (opposite) only physiological saline was injected.

4.7 HEALING ASSESSMENT

Research into scarring is still in its infancy. Morris, in 1997, described a study in rabbit ears to evaluate the treatment of hypertrophic scarring with trioncinolone compared to saline solution

(Morris DE, Wu L, Zhao LL, et al, 1997).

Historically, the way to assess human scarring has been through clinical studies. This requires a scar assessment tool that is defined in a common medical language. The Vancouver scale has been widely accepted and is most commonly used for burns (Sullivan T, Smith J, Kermode J, et al, 1990; Baryza MJ, Baryza GA, 1995; Nedelec B, Shankowsky A, Tredgett EE, 2000; Mustoe TA, Cooter RD, Gold MH, et al, 2002). In 1998, Beausang expanded this scale, making it more complete for assessing linear scars after surgery or trauma (Beausang E, Floyd H, Dunn KW, et al, 1998). As these two scales did not consider the component, Draaijers made modifications creating a scale that depends on the assessment of the patient and the observer (Draaijers LJ, Tempelman FRH, Botman YAM, et al, 2004). In addition to these scales, morphometric assessment using digital photography has been considered as a method of documenting and assessing scars (Davey RB, Sprod RT, Neild TO, 1999).In this study, scars were assessed using the following methods:

1. Patient/observer scales (Draaijers LJ, Tempelman FRH, Botman YAM, et al, 2004). It consists of two numerical scales validated and tested against the Vancouver scale (Sullivan T, Smith J, Kermode J, et al, 1990; Baryza MJ, Baryza GA, 1995; Nedelec B, Shankowsky A, Tredgett EE, 2000; Mustoe TA, Cooter RD, Gold MH, et al, 2002). The observer scale contains five evaluation items: vascularisation, pigmentation, elasticity, thickness and relief (Appendix C). The patient scale contains six evaluation items: colour, elasticity, thickness, relief, itching and pain (Appendix D). Each evaluation item has a score ranging from 1 to 10, with a score of 10 meaning the worst scar and the worst sensation imaginable. The sum of the observer's scale scores ranges from 5 to 50, while the sum of the patient's scores ranges from 6 to 60. The lowest score sums, 5 and 6 respectively, reflect normal skin (Appendix E).

   - Four observers, one of whom was the patient herself, assessed the healing results at 1, 2, 3, 4, 5, 6 and 12 months. Two plastic surgeons and a dermatologist were appointed as medical observers, all with more than 10 years of specialisation and not belonging to the clinical staff of the São Lucas Hospital at PUCRS.

2. Morphometric scaling by digital photography and image analysis (Image Pro Plus, Media Cybernetics, Silver Spring, MD, USA) (Davey RB, Sprod RT, Neild TO, 1999).

- Photographic documentation was carried out with the help of a hydraulic tube (made of PVC), on which the camera was supported. The tube was used for two purposes: to avoid dispersing the light from the flash, which was activated in all the photos, and to keep the same distance from all the documented patients (Figure 13).

- The photometric evaluation was carried out by a doctor from the Plastic Surgery Department of the São Lucas Hospital of the PUCRS, who was unaware of the sides on which the adult adipose tissue stem cells were implanted.

- The scar was assessed by the Optical Image Density (OID) by averaging the perpendicular length of the scar at ten points, on both sides, at the adult adipose tissue stem cell implantation sites and in the control.

- All the patients surveyed were photographed during all the assessment phases with the same camera (SONY®: DSC-W7, 7.2 mega pixels), the same lighting and distance.

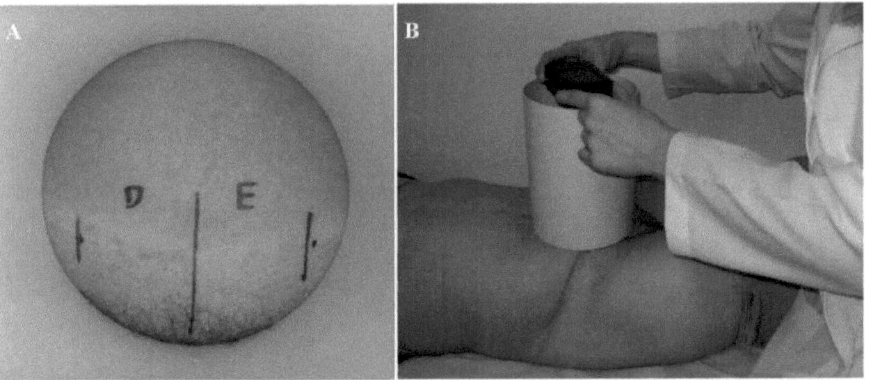

Figure 13 - Photographic documentation: The camera is supported by a PVC hydraulic tube. A)

suprapubic photography; B) patient being photographed.

4.8 STATISTICAL ANALYSIS

All the elements observed in the patients were quantified by analysing the pixels in the photographs or by scoring the patients' impressions and the doctors' assessments. Descriptive measures were obtained by mean and standard deviation at each assessment point. Areas under the curve were then calculated for the points formed by the two sides of the scar to be compared. The curves were compared using Student's t-test for paired samples. Next, the proportion of observations that were favourable and unfavourable to the stem cell intervention were also compared using theBinomial test. The significance level adopted was alpha=0.05. The data was analysed by intention to treat using the LOCF (Last Obs. Carried Forward) protocol, processed and analysed using the SPSS software, version 15.0.

4.8.1 Sample size

Based on an initial expectation of a moderate to large impact of the intervention, we estimated that the magnitude of the effect would be 0.85 standard deviation units in the evaluation scores. We therefore determined that at least 15 pairs of observations would be needed to achieve a statistical power of 90% at a significance level of 5%.

4.9 ETHICAL ASPECTS

This research has been approved:

On 22/08/2005, by the Coordinating Committee of the Postgraduate Programme in Medicine and Health Sciences at PUCRS, Protocol no.° 264/05-PG (Annex A).

On 24/11/2005, by the Ethics Committee of the São Lucas Hospital of the Pontifical Catholic University of Rio Grande do Sul - PUCRS, Protocol no. 05/02789 (Annex B).

All the patients who took part in this study signed the "Informed Consent Form".

CHAPTER 5

RESULTS

A total of 18 patients underwent surgery, of whom 17 (94.4%) had excellent or good results and 1 (5.5%) was considered to have a poor result because there was dehiscence in the suture in the suprapubic region. A further 5 patients dropped out during the course of the study (27.7%), with 12 remaining until the end (66.6%). Using the Draaijers Scale criteria (Draaijers LJ, Tempelman FRH, Botman YAM, et al, 2004), it was possible to verify that the sides implanted with adult adipose tissue stem cells showed better healing than those (control) where only saline was infiltrated (Figures 14 and 15).

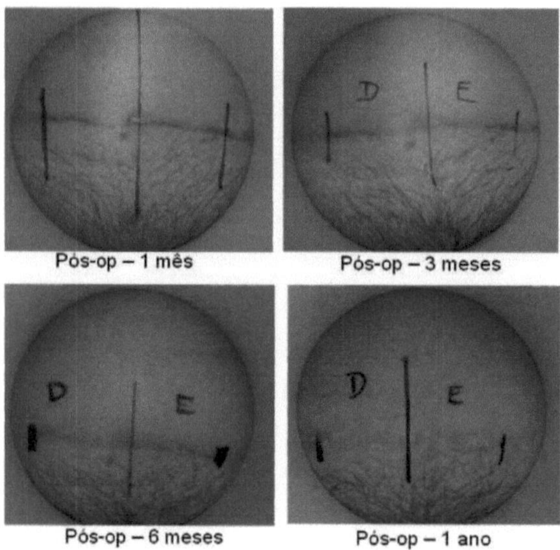

Figura 14   - Implantation of adult stem cells from adipose tissue on the right side. Results.

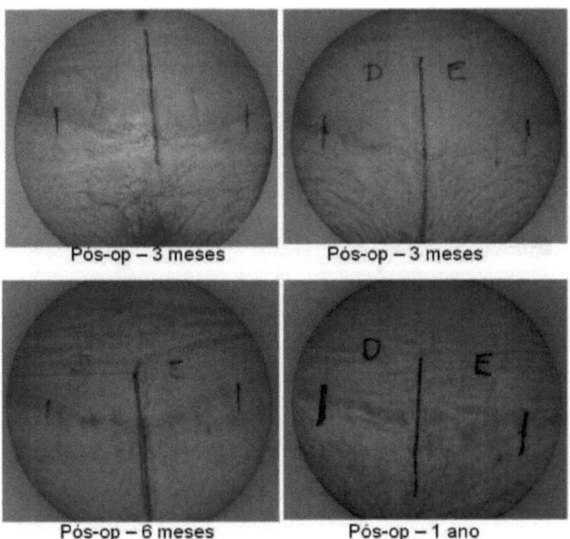

Figura 15   - Implantation of adult stem cells from adipose tissue on the <u>left</u> side. Results

When comparing the photometric aspects, no statistically significant difference was detected in the random measurement (P=0.44) or in the total measurement (P=0.66).

To compare the patients' evaluations, 6 aspects were considered (pain, itching, colour, stiffness, thickness and irregularity). None of these were found to be statistically significant (P>0.17) when analysing the scores. However, considering all the evaluation events over the observation period, 42 measurement points were obtained. Of these, 15 were in favour of the control and 27 in favour of the stem cells, which reached a significance level of P = 0.12 in favour of the stem cell intervention.In the medical observers' assessment, 5 aspects were considered (vascularisation, pigmentation, thickness, contracture and elasticity). None of the

of these aspects, a statistically significant difference was found (P>0.37). However, when considering the distribution of evaluations over the observation period, 35 measurement points were obtained. Of these, 8 were in favour of the control and 27 in favour of the stem cells, which reached a significance level of P = 0.003 in favour of the stem cell intervention (Figure 16).

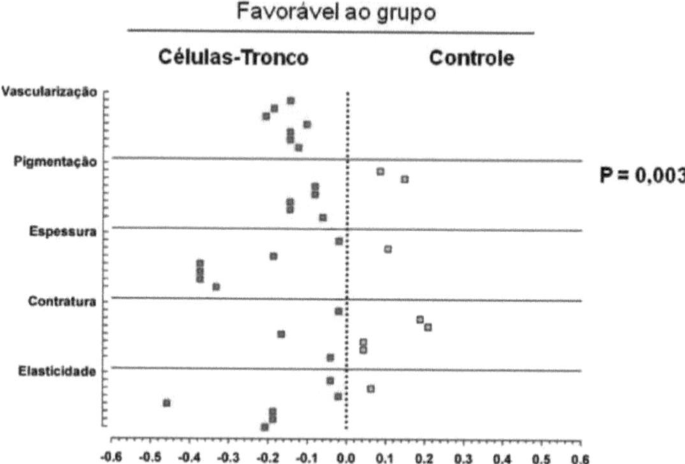

Figura 16   - Evaluation by doctors: Scatter plot of points representing the distribution of evaluation events over the observation period (P=0.003).

When evaluations were stratified by patients and photometry, no significance was found, probably due to the small number of events evaluated; however, considering all the evaluations carried out (doctors, patients and photometry), a statistically significant difference was found in favour of implantation with adult adipose tissue stem cells, p<0.001 (Table 1).

Table 1 - Comparison of evaluation events during the observation period

Aspect in evaluation	Events evaluation	Favourable to the group		P
		Cells Trunk	Control	
Photometric	**14**	11	3	0,106
Patients	**42**	27	15	0,120
Doctors	**35**	27	8	0,003
Total	**91**	65	26	**<0,001**

It can be seen that out of a total of 91 events, 65 were in favour of the stem cell implant and 26 in favour of the control (P<0.001).

CHAPTER 6

DISCUSSION

The results of abdominoplasty are secondary to the focus of this study, which exclusively analyses skin healing. However, they are important for proving that carrying out this study did not cause any alterations that could compromise the post-operative evolution and results of the participating patients.

Evidence-based procedures (Ativeh BS, 2007) are used to ensure good post-surgical healing. In addition to a refined surgical technique and care to position the scars in accordance with the skin's lines of force, any tension on the suture lines should be avoided. In the post-operative period, immobilisation and compression of the scar is recommended, including during the maturation phase (Lorenz PA, Longaker MT, 2006).

Therapeutic measures such as corticosteroids, botulinum toxin, vitamins A and E, silicone adhesive tapes, laser and radiotherapy are used to prevent hypertrophic scars or keloids (Lorenz PA, Longaker MT, 2006; Xiao Z, Zhang F, Cui Z, 2009; Horswell BB, 1998; Viera MH, Amini S, Barman B, 2009; HaedersdalM, Moreau KE, Beyer DM, Nymann P, Alsbj0rn, 2009). This randomised controlled study was carried out with the same objectives, aiming to improve scarring. The implantation of adult adipose tissue stem cells in the dermis of the abdominoplasty surgical wound showed a beneficial effect on healing. The cells used were autologous, had no contraindications and did not cause side effects, as can occur in other procedures using corticosteroids or radiotherapy.

It was not possible to carry out a comparative analysis with other similar studies due to the scarcity of published research evaluating the implantation of adult stem cells from adipose tissue in surgical incisions in human skin. The studies we did find analysed this in laboratory animals (Stoff A et al, 2009; Saton H et al, 2009) and their results, as well as those of this study, refer to the beneficial effects of cell therapy on skin healing.

As this is an initial study, the results reported here can be considered promising when compared with research that has been carried out for longer, such as experiments using cell therapy to regenerate other tissues. Studies into pathologies or trauma to organs such as the heart, liver, kidney and peripheral nerves (Mays RW et al, 2007; Navarro-Alvarez N, Soto-Gutierrez A, Kobavashi, 2009; Watorek E, Klinger M, 2009; Braga-Silva J et al, 2008) have proven that their tissues can be regenerated.

CHAPTER 7

CONCLUSION

The results of skin healing in a post-operative abdominoplasty wound after the implantation of adult stem cells derived from adipose tissue were satisfactory.

REFERENCES

Adzick NS, Longaker MT: Fetal wound healing. New York, Chapman & Hall, 1992.

Ativeh BS. Nonsurgical management of hypertrophic scars: evidence-based therapies, standard practices, and emerging methods. 31(5): 468-92; discussion 4934. Aesthetic Plast Surg. 2007.

Baryza MJ, Baryza GA. The Vancouver scar scale: an administration tool and its interrater reability. J Burn Care Rehabil 16:535, 1995.

Beausang E, Floyd H, Dunn KW, et al. A new quantitative scale for clinical scar assessment. Plast Reconst Surg 102:1954-1961,1998.

Braga-Silva J, Gehlen D, Padoin AV, Machado DC, Garicochea B, Costa da Costa J. Can local supply of bone marrow mononuclear cells improve the outcome from late tubulalar repair of human median and ulnar nerves? J Hand Surg (BR). 2008, in press.

Bullard M, Cass D, Adzick N, Banda M. TGF-beta1 decreases interstitial collagenase in healing human foetal skin. Surg Forum 47:762-764, 1996.

Daley GQ, Goodell MA, Snyder EY. Realistic prospects for stem cell therapeutics. Haematology. 398-418, 2003.

Davey RB, Sprod RT, Neild TO. Computerised colour: a technique for the assessment of burn scar hypertrophy. A preliminary report. Burns 25:207, 1999.

De Ugarte DA, Morizono K, Elbarbar A, et al. Comparison of multi-lineage cells from human adipose tissue and bone marrow. Cells Tissues Organs. 174: 101-9, 2003.

Draaijers LJ, Tempelman FRH, Botman YAM, et al. The patient and observer scar assessment scale: a reliable and feasible tool for scar evaluation. Plast Reconst Surg 113:1960-1965, 2004.

Estes JM, Vande Berg JS, Adzick NS, et al. Phenotypic and functional features of myofibroblasts in sheep foetal wounds. Differentiation 56:173-181, 1994

Fodor WL. Tissue engineering and cell based therapies, from the bench to the clinic: The potential to replace, repair and regenerate. Reproductive Biology and Endocrinology. 1, 1-6, 2003.

Fournier P. Lipodissection in body sculpturing: The dry procedure. Plast. Reconstr. Surg. 1983; 72: 598.

Fraser JK, Wulur I, Alfonso Z, Hedrick MH. Fat tissue: an underappreciated source of stem cells for biotechnology. Trends Biotechnol. 2006; 24: 150-4.

HaedersdalM, Moreau KE, Beyer DM, Nymann P, Alsbj0rn. Fractional nanabalative 1540 nm laser resurfacing for thermal burn scars: a randomised controlled trial. 41(3):189-95. Lasers Surg Med. 2009.

Horswell BB. Scar modification. Techniques for revision and camouflage. 6(2): Atlas Oral Maxillofac Surg Clin North Am. 1998.

Illouz YG. A new method for localised lipodystrophies. Rev. Chir. Esthet. 1980; 4: 19 (6).

Lambert APFandonai AF, Bonatto D, Machado DC, Henriques JAP. Differentiation of human adipose-derived adult stem cells into neuronal tissue: Does it work? Differentiation (2009), doi: 10.1016/j.diff.2008.10. 10.016.

Lin R, Sullivan K, Argenta P, et al. Scarless human fetal skin repair is intrinsic to the fetal fibroblast and occurs in the absence of an inflammatory response: In situ hybridisation and immunohistochemical studies. Wound Repair Regen 2:297, 1994.

Loeffler M Bratke T, Paulus U, Clonality and life cycles of intestinal crypts explained by a dependent stochastic model of epithelial stemoganisation. J. Theor Biol. 186, 41-54, 1997.

Lorenz PA, Longaker MT: Wound Healing: Repair Biology and Wound and Scar Treatment. In Mathes, Plastic Surgery Vol. 1, Chapter 11, Saunders - Elsevier - 2006.

Martinez-Estrada OM, Munoz-Santos Y, Julve J, et al. Human adipose tissue as a source of Flk-1[+] cells: new method of differentiation and expansion. Cardiovasc Res 65(2):328-333, 2005.

Mays RW, van't Hof W, Ting AE, Perry R, Deans R. Development of adult pluripotent stem cell therapies for ischemic injury and disease. 7(2):173-84. Expert Opin Biol Ther. 2007. Joggers SJ, Hatzop.

Morris DE, Wu L, Zhao LL, et al. Acute and chronic animal models for excessive dermal scarring: quantitative studies. Plast Reconst Surg 100:674-681, 1997.

Mustoe TA, Cooter RD, Gold MH, et al. International clinical recommendations on scar management. Plast Reconst Surg 110:560-571, 2002.

Navarro-Alvarez N, Soto-Gutierrez A, Kobavashi. Stem Cell research and therapy for liver. 4(2): 141-6.Curr Stem Cell Res Ther. 2009.

Nedelec B, Shankowsky A, Tredgett EE. Rating the resolving hypertrophic scar: comparison of the Vancouver scar scale and scar volume. J Burn Care Rehabil 21:205, 2000.

Padoin AV, Braga-Silva J, Martins P, et al. Sources of Processed Lipoaspirate: Influence of Donor Site on Cell Concentration. Plast Reconst Surg Aug-2008: 61618.

Pitanguy I. Abdominoplasty. In Aest Palst Surg of Head and Body, Chap 2:99-116. Springer-Verlag, 1981.

Pitman GH. Liposuction at Boby Contourig. In Grabb and Smith's Plastic Surgery, Chap 54:669-91. Ffth Ed. Lippincott-Raven - 1997).

Pittenger MF, Mackay AM, Beck SC et al. Multilineage potential of adult human mesenchymal stem cells. Science. 284, 143-147, 1999.

Pontes R. Abdominoplasty - En bloc resection and its application in thigh *lift* and torsoplasty. Rio de Janeiro, Revinter, 2004.

Porter R: The Greatest benefit to mankind, a medical history of humanity. New York, WWNorton, 1997.

Sabiston Textbook of Surgery: The biological basis of modern surgical practice. 17th Edition. Philadelphia, Elsevier, 2004.

Safford KM, Hicok KC, Safford SD, et al. Neurogenic differentiation of murine and human adipose-derived stromal cells. Biochemical and Biophysical Res Com 294:371- 379, 2002.

Saton H, Kishi K, Tanaka Y, Nakajima T, Akasaka Y, Ishii T. Transplanted Mesenchymal stem cells are effective for skin regeneration in acute cutaneous wounds. 18(4):362-9. Exp Dermatol. 2009.

Sinder R. Abdominoplasties. In Carreirão S, Cardin V, Goldenberg D. Plastic Surgery. Atheneu, 2005.

Stoff A, Rivera AA, Sanjib Banerjee N, Moore ST, Michel Numnum T, Espinosa-de- Los-Monteros A, Richter DF, Siegal GP, Chow LT, Fedman D, Vasconez LO, Michael

Mathis J, Stoff-Khalili MA, Curiel DT. Promotion of incisional wound repair by human mesenchymal stem cell transplantation. 18(4):362-9. Exp Dermatol. 2009

Sullivan T, Smith J, Kermode J, et al. Rating the burn scar. J Burn Care Rehabil 11:256, 1990.

Tohill M, Terenghi G. Stem-cell plasticity and therapy for injuries of the peripheral nervous system. Biotechnology and Applied Biochemistry. 40, 17-24, 2004.

Tuan RS, Boland G, Tuli R. Adult mesenchymal stem cells and cell-based tissue engineering Research Arthritis & Therapy. 5, 32-45, 2003.

Vasconez LO, De La Torre JI. Abdominoplasty. In Mathes, Plastic Surgery Vol. 6, Chapter 11, Saunders - Elsevier - 2006.

Viera MH, Amini S, Barman B. Do postsurgical interventions optimise ultimate scar cosmesis. 144(3): 243-57. G Ital Dermatol Venereol. 2009.

Watorek E, Klinger M. Stem cells in nephrology: present status and future. 54(1):45-50. Arch Immunol Ther Exp (Warsz). 2009.

Xiao Z, Zhang F, Cui Z. Treatment of hypertrophic scars with intralesional botulinum toxin type a injections: a preliminary report. 33(3): 409-12. Aesthetic Plast Surg. 2009.

Zuk PA, Zhu M, Mizumo H, et al. Multi lineage cells from adipose tissue: implications for cell-based therapies. Tissue Eng. 7:211-28, 2003.

Annex A - Letter of approval of the Research Protocol by the Coordinating Committee of the

Postgraduate Programme in Medicine and Health Sciences at PUCRS

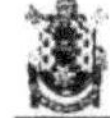 PONTIFÍCIA UNIVERSIDADE CATÓLICA DO RIO GRANDE DO SUL
FACULDADE DE MEDICINA
PÓS-GRADUAÇÃO EM MEDICINA 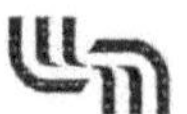

264/05-PG

Porto Alegre, 22 de agosto de 2005.

Ao Professor
Pedro Djacir Escobar Martins
N/Faculdade

Prezado Professor :

Comunicamos que a proposta de tese intitulada "Estudo do implante de células tronco adultas do tecido adiposo na cicatrização da pele em ferida pós-operatória de abdominoplastia" foi aprovada pela Comissão Coordenadora do Programa de Pós-Graduação em Medicina e Ciências da Saúde.

Informamos que a mesma deve ser encaminhada ao comitê de Ética em Pesquisa, através do CINAPE, 2º andar do HSL, ramal 2687. Em anexo, cópia da avaliação.

Atenciosamente,

Profa. Dra. Magda Lahorgue Nunes
Coordenadora do Programa de Pós-Graduação
em Medicina e Ciências da Saúde

C/c: Prof. Dr. Jefferson Luis Braga da Silva
Profa. Dra. Denise Cantarelli Machado

Av. Ipiranga, 6690 - 3º andar
Caixa Postal - 1429
CEP 90610-000- Porto Alegre - RS - Brasil

Fone: 0 (xx) 51 3320-3318
Fax: 0 (xx) 51 3320-3852
e-mail: medicina-pg@pucrs.br

Annex B - Letter of approval of the Research Protocol by the PUCRS Ethics Committee

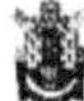 PONTIFÍCIA UNIVERSIDADE CATÓLICA DO RIO GRANDE DO SUL
PRÓ-REITORIA DE PESQUISA E PÓS-GRADUAÇÃO
COMITÊ DE ÉTICA EM PESQUISA - CEP - PUCRS 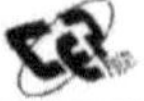

Ofício nº 1130/05-CEP   Porto Alegre, 24 de novembro de 2005.

Senhor(a) Pesquisador(a):

O Comitê de Ética em Pesquisa da PUCRS apreciou e aprovou seu protocolo de pesquisa intitulado: "Estudo do implante de células tronco adultas do tecido adiposo na cicatrização da pele em ferida pós-operatória de abdominoplastia".

Sua investigação está autorizada a partir da presente data.

Atenciosamente,

Prof. Dr. Caio Coelho Marques
COORDENADOR EM EXERCÍCIO

Ilmo(a) Sr(a)
Dr(a) Denise Cantarelli Machado
N/Universidade

Appendix C - Draaijers Scale - Observer

OBSERVER SCALE (Draaijers,2004)[36] .

DATA: _______   PACIENTE: ________________   OSERVADOR: _______________

LADO DIREITO		LADO ESQUERDO	
Vascularização	□ □ □ □ □ □ □ □ □	Vascularização	□ □ □ □ □ □ □ □ □
Pigmentação	□ □ □ □ □ □ □ □ □	Pigmentação	□ □ □ □ □ □ □ □ □
Espessura	□ □ □ □ □ □ □ □ □	Espessura	□ □ □ □ □ □ □ □ □
Contraste	□ □ □ □ □ □ □ □ □	Contraste	□ □ □ □ □ □ □ □ □
Elasticidade	□ □ □ □ □ □ □ □ □	Elasticidade	□ □ □ □ □ □ □ □ □

Pele normal   1 2 3 4 5 6 7 8 9 10   Pior cicatriz   Pele normal   1 2 3 4 5 6 7 8 9 10   Pior cicatriz

Annex D - Draaijers Scale - Patient

PATIENT SCALE (Draaijers, 2004)[36]

DATA: _______   PACIENTE: ________________

LADO DIREITO		LADO ESQUERDO	
A cicatriz é dolorida?	□ □ □ □ □ □ □ □ □	A cicatriz é dolorida?	□ □ □ □ □ □ □ □ □
A cicatriz coça?	□ □ □ □ □ □ □ □ □	A cicatriz coça?	□ □ □ □ □ □ □ □ □
A cor da cicatriz está diferente?	□ □ □ □ □ □ □ □ □	A cor da cicatriz está diferente?	□ □ □ □ □ □ □ □ □
A cicatriz está mais endurecida?	□ □ □ □ □ □ □ □ □	A cicatriz está mais endurecida?	□ □ □ □ □ □ □ □ □
A espessura está diferente?	□ □ □ □ □ □ □ □ □	A espessura está diferente?	□ □ □ □ □ □ □ □ □
A cicatriz está irregular?	□ □ □ □ □ □ □ □ □	A cicatriz está irregular?	□ □ □ □ □ □ □ □ □

Não   1 2 3 4 5 6 7 8 9 10   Sim   Não   1 2 3 4 5 6 7 8 9 10   Sim

Annex E - Evaluation criteria

<u>ASSESSMENT CRITERIA</u>

Vascularização   Normal   -   Rosa   -   Vermelho -   Roxo

Pigmentação   Normal   -   Hipo   -   Mixta   -   Hiper

Espessura   Plana   -   < 2mm   -   2 a 5mm   - > 5mm

Contraste   Sem contraste   -   Pouco -   Muito contraste

Elasticidade   Normal   -   Firme -   Dura   -   Contratura

Pele   normal   **1**   **2**   **3**   **4**   **5**   **6**   **7**   **8**   **9**   **10**   **Pior   cicatriz**

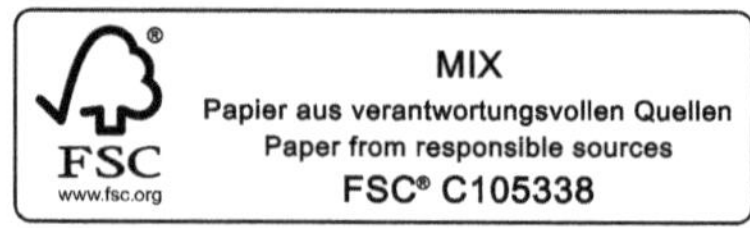

Printed by Books on Demand GmbH, Norderstedt / Germany